MW01487709

BONES
AWAITING
THE
BLAZE

TIFFANY ELLIOTT

AN INLANDIA INSTITUTE PUBLICATION

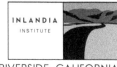

INLANDIA
INSTITUTE

RIVERSIDE, CALIFORNIA

Bones Awaiting The Blaze
Copyright © 2022 by Tiffany Elliott

ISBN: 978-1-955969-26-0 (paperback)

Cover art, book design and layout: Mark Givens
Printed and bound in the United States
Distributed by Ingram

Library of Congress Control Number: 2024931905

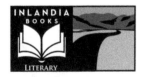

Published by Inlandia Institute
Riverside, California
www.InlandiaInstitute.org
First Edition

Bones Awaiting The Blaze

Tiffany Elliott

CONTENTS

I twist a helix upon myself
the crookedness smoothed into planes
I can slide through. I read
about the work of CRISPR geneticists
in the news and wonder
how much would be left if all traces
of you were excised, held in my palm
the way you held my leg,
writhing against my grip
as I against yours, breaking
as you broke me. An eggshell pierced—
bacteria a river twisting
the yolk into green shining
on the banks outside our home.
Is this what you meant when you told me
I must honor, that God demanded my honor
of you? I look through shrouded eyes
behold God's countenance. Sunlight
can purify, but anyone who's taken
basic biology can tell you:
It also corrupts.

I want to swallow my sewing machine, needle by needle, unbinding the gears, a
    thimble sticking in my craw, the thread a delicate noose

the way I learned sewing was for girls with ribbons in their braids whose button-eyed
    dolls matryoshka womanhood. Grasp the needle and pull

to unfurl the perfected stitch, to let their black eyes roll along woodgrain floors and
    out the door. I want to

sew penises on the Ken doll's misshapen groin, line him up in a row, pluck
the blue eyes at the root, the orbits gone glassy, swallow them all in turn, one by one.

The doll traveled steerage
in great-grandmother's
satchel, lovingly knit beaded net
for her hair, headscarf
shielding. The painted
pucker, winged eye
a butterfly. Few Hungarian
words remain. Goulash and paprikash
its red staining our pot
the onions with skins on for color
and flavor. The doll reproves, haughty
half-smirking: she knows
I have lost the thread.

The Owl

Outside the window,
the orange grove blossoms its scent

through the warm evening air and
an owl sits on the wooden post, watching

over dad's car, lights off,
bumping over dirt road potholes

The engine revs as he rounds the corner,
headlights now lurching, slicing

through the pepper tree
shadow branches. I cry for mom

to wind the box again and prove
that it still works, though I fear the spring is

weakening, breaking. Her eyes can't focus
on the moonlit yard. *Do you hear it*, I ask,

as the music box winds down one last time.

My tongue unravels curse words, slurps
soapy bubbles from the toilet
and squirts them into a Dawn bottle.
Dad's hands are magical—they remove
fingerprints from my legs as tears frog-crawl
backward through craterous ducts. My jaw
unclamps, my fingers
unplug ears which uncatch
my mother's drawling drunken words,
and she unswills the vodka
pouring into the Smirnoff bottle
like a baptismal font.

I wrap her belly
with my arms,

feel for the
cracks, watch her

at bathtime to see
how she takes herself off,

layer by layer, to
unstitch her arms from

their sockets, to unbuckle
at her navel. I crawl inside

her chasmic form
that swallows, the guts

reaching, the intestines
roping my wrist.

Come home, they croon,
and I span her with my arms.

doesn't have a face. He chases me through the hallway and into my bedroom, where all the floorboards but one are gone, and in the cavern below a hundred arms with their hundred hands reach. When I fall into them, the tickling wakes me up, and I tell my mother I had a nightmare. She says she knows I am lying

because she heard laughter. I look back, wonder how she didn't understand the duplicity, remember the day she tickled and tickled and tickled me, laughing at my struggle until I peed.

beautiful, sinews strapping
arms like spindles with threads
with threats, locks limply obscuring
the marble glasses of eyes
a frowzy deposit frowning
down the lips, parted wide
strawberry inside a strong tongue
tasting treats, she waited and sated
your hunger, the roof of your mouth
tingles, her mud mixed
in a sour patch, lift the latch
find the house, its candy shingles
its raspberry roughness, its fried
dough door beckons. Her claw
a nail-heavy thing reaching—

Let's say the sky was blue that day instead of grey. Let's say the dark part of the moon was full and smiling. Let's say your smile crinkled and cracked when I told a joke, and I held that joke in my hand and put it into my journal that night. Let's say I reread that page over and over for the next week and my smile matched yours, but lumpy in bits where yours was smooth. Let's say we tried to count the stars and only made it to fifty-seven before dissolving into giggles like the little girls we should have been. Let's say your arms held me and mine held you, and we were sisters. Let's say this was every day, and every night we went to sleep in lumpy blankets knit with strawberries on them by grandma. Let's say we loved each other and turned the night into day.

Does glass remember
its ancestry, blown
in waves over the Savannah or
trussed by turtles
egging the future
in pits. Curling the single hairy
root of a palm, does sand
question starlight—
so distant
from the burning
that transforms. Do stars
peek our moon
longing her weightless
embrace. I search those same
stars divining
the way a lifeline flows
through rivers and into
the Salton Sea fifty miles
from a buried
teacup shard where
you whispered
I will return
someday. And in slanting
May sunlight, you
stand on Indian clay
north of the ravine, my
name floating the orange
scent of all the late blossoms
I will never pluck again.

I cover you in ink, the flavor harsh
on my eardrum. I eat words
ten syllables at once as we fuck
atop stacks of forbidden newsprint.

I spell you in grease
between the library stacks, the stains
Rorschach images of birds, of vines,
of mice that notch books, of their feces,
of tulips pressed between
pages—they had their time,
they shed petals one by one
like woodlice.

I have two words left. I lock them
away behind my bared teeth.

find a word that slathers   your tongue   in light
pop it red and yellow   sing a rainbow   make me feel how
        an oil slick   invades   and cross
the moat   filled to leaking   whistle for me
        you hold photons   then eat a sunset   give to me and
I'll choke   on the river   of them

do not laugh   –   join me

covalent, our bonds
        are loaded weapons,
the chemistry reactive

pairing. A woman once
        said *to be perfected*
you must hold together

like a tapestry, like
        the electrons
between our

bodies. Years ago,
        I swore off
chemistry, the flask

of your hands,
        traded them in
for a crucible, set the

burner's flame blue
        charred all the cells
you left on me

to dust.

Ophiocordyceps unilateralis famously uses a specific species of ant to complete its life cycle. To live, it must zombify an ant.

—Kyle Hill, *Scientific American*

You, lover, were a cordyceps
        dream, hot on
            the back of my
    neck with your
            uninvited spore
rare and working
        under my backplate.
            I cannot resist
    your zombie
            charms, your
mimicry arms
            engulfing
        enfolding. I climb
            the highest branch
together, lover, as your
        essence fills every
                crevice
        of my stacked
            carapace, twilight
musk seeping from
        my pores, ecstasy in
                the perfumed air.
            Spring is all around this
exoskeleton that
        blooms with
                the fullness of you.

My face is full of desert sands, hollows
shading the eyes except at noon
under the supraorbital ridge
lined with cacti that shake
with subcutaneous tarantulas.

Those spiders, no respect
for personal space, divide the lashes.
Swallow the dishes woven from
my fringe—it is all the food they have
to give. Inside, one bowl fills another,
cupboards stacked to the diaphragm
clattering at each cough. Move carefully.

If they fall, I'll reach
through the esophagus,
straighten the stacks, brush
a broom across my back to clear
cobwebs and the mess.

No one said this was going to be pretty.

my arms the rags of them that flail in winds, you cannot have my legs or the joints, cannot pull me apart at the seams to find my shelled core

I fold my heart, tuck it into your sleep
can't you see I had nothing to give
I pull at threads on your shoulder do not leave me
I pluck a blue button an eye

love me love me, can't you see the cord I fashioned you I pieced my own threads together, can you bear it as I once bore you, do not leave me

I say I can't be your daughter
anymore. I try to make this
about you, about how

you fragmented
me from our family
dying for love

even after you and I sat
in the dean's mahogany
office and you lied:

Of course she
can live with me
what kind of a mother

do you think I am.
What I never say is
this is about me,

no clue where
I am. And this is
about when I was ten

and asked *do you love me*
as the barren
branches of an ill-

planned plum tree knocked
fruitlessly at the window
and I waited for you

with your loosely
hanging drunken skin
to say that my sister,

at least, cleaned her room
thoroughly. This is
about my final

essay for Medieval Lit
composed on
the Heroic Christ in

two-sentence chunks—Christ
in peril, Christ the objectified
hero, Christ as Rood, Christ as

lover, Christ as mother
—until the morning
before my paper was due

and the only words I
could think were
the bitter ones you said

in my car on Interstate 395
after visiting your
brother recovering from

three new stents, and he
handed you his iPhone
with instructions: *Talk*

to your sister—she hadn't
heard your voice since
you quit your job

and let me pay your bills. Ice
cream cools your cookie and
stillness is plated between us

as I wait to see if you
will be the first to stand, to
walk away, the cacophonous din

of knives scraping tin and
glass carafes chink
empty spots on the sidebars

throwing caramel rainbows
over patrons and
over us.

When my sweat beaded on my lip as it
almost parted, almost asked you to stay
in the booth with cracked red vinyl
seat backs and varnish peeling a roadmap
around your salad. I explore
a mahogany office and wonder
is this the office you remember, or
was the burgundy tapestry royal blue, was
there a window, and did the dean
leaning back in the black oiled leather have
a mustache or was it his bare lip
that trembled. Drop of water
about to plummet into the porcelain sink,
and in that moment, two drops
and two sinks, one aluminum and one
pale pink, one drop water
and another blood. Who can say
if it was really water anyway, when
the dean left us and the wall clock with its
twinned weights hung over our heads
then dropped into a filled lake. Who can say
if you're right, if the pendulum
swung your way or knocked me
off balance. The only evidence I have
is a water-stained journal,
fear that pitted my stomach
when I forgave the man
who was beating me, and
sweat rolling when you left
in a rage and forgot your pizza
in the brown box, and for once
I didn't call out reminding you to take it.

In a shallow pit all of her
that was left asked, *Give me*
what left the stain browning the base
I can't remember everything
we could have had, the glass still
on a shelf, and I gave
the natural pucker of her lips
amber honey to drown. I asked
for the tip of an apology, handed
her a lemon, green-edged
and out of reach.

Sitting high on a sill, she asks for a glass of water.

Out of reach, I handed her
a lemon, green-edged on the tip
of an apology. I asked for
amber honey to drown the natural
pucker of her lips growing
with everything we could have had
The glass is still on a shelf
and I can't remember
what left the stain browning
the base. *Give me* she asked
and I gave all of her that was
left in the shallow pit

"This place is going to burn just like we planned"

Text message from the man who started a 2018 fire that burned 23,136 acres in the Cleveland National Forest in Southern CA

i.

A cloth soaked with linseed oil
will turn itself gradually dark

as the chemical reaction
spontaneously combusts

—

the rag my mother used to oil
her butcher block almost set

her home ablaze the sooty
smoke tendrils rising off lint

an incensed prayer a foreboding
fear as a mile away

the riverbottom burned

—

rumors it was a controlled fire set by police to remove the homeless
from the Santa Ana River Trail encampment consumed us all

ii.

Last year, a man
I never met

set the world under a
magnificent glass

they said the wind
tasted tin and the linger

of new charcoal
in the days before fire

painted our skyline brown
camo underpants in hand

he streaked through town
said to all who would listen

I can read your thoughts

he fondled dry brush, held it up
lace against the sun, whispered

I will return you to the burning

iii.

Mental health workers are prohibited from revealing whether a
person is receiving or has received mental health services, unless
a proper release of information form is completed. That said,
many state laws have been altered to provide better and more
comprehensive services. Notably, major changes were instituted
after multiple families lost loved ones to suicide, despite warnings
to mental health professionals. If a person is reported to have made
a suicidal or homicidal threat, CA state laws mandate that proper
authorities must be contacted to prevent harm to the individual or
to others. This is called "duty to warn."

There is no such duty for fire safety personnel.

iv.

I held my mother's
hand like a cup

I could not drink from
spilled warm breath

on lacquered wood
where is she

I ran from
her smoking fingers

did we do all this just
to see our world burn

or was she
overwrought

a dry stem inching
toward her own flame

v.

An August 2018 Washington Post article
reported that a local man had been flagging
problems with the suspected Holy Fire arsonist
for the past three years.

It's very sad

I agree, Public Affairs Liaison Walker, sadness
is something we share in a small

burning part of this country

Supervisor Spitzer is also sad,
The community is angry and sad, he says,
and also, that he wasn't made aware of the threats

Passive voice
because in times of crisis, no one wants to say

I dropped the ball or My department's communication
with other departments was inadequate

Or We should have done better

vi.

Commandment

a child is never commanded
to love its parents

a woman is never commanded
to love her husband

why do all God's plans leave me ashes
scented on the wind
the remains of a doll hand-sewn and discarded

a pastor once said it is in a woman's nature to love
and it is in a child's nature to love unconditionally

I burn with love
all my stuffing eked out in stages
in plumes of smoke

I ask God why and God never answers

a pastor once said God always answers
our most burning questions and another pastor said
God never will

if I place this rag doll on a funeral pyre
will God accept as a sacrifice
its putrid smoke

my mother won't pull it from the flames
hold it to her chest
sing sweet lullabies in alto tones

I swallow all the questions I never meant to pose

it is too late to stop the spread of fire
stop the winds spreading ash
stop the idle hands
stop sparks

I stand before my mother
ask God what is commanded of me

there is a stillness in burning that is not silent
while the bush watches and waits
before it is consumed

I ask God for revelation
burning sword tongues of fire
stillness beneath the winds

and interpret the stillness as answer

vii.

Catalogue of images of the Holy Fire in Lake Elsinore:

August 8: Airplane dropping foam behind evacuated houses

August 8: A resident loading belongings into a truck

August 8: A home burning

August 9: A lone boat floating on Lake Mission Viejo

August 9: A sheriff's deputy standing guard outside a gate leading to the
    forest

August 9: A firefighter helplessly watching the blaze

August 9: Homes burning

viii.

I fall out of love
over and over with
you, you
of flower stems

that branch from
us, bones

awaiting the blaze.

for buttons I
swallowed like

robin's eggs when
I was young, hoping

to hatch a doll
under my skin

a ribbon for hair
curls unfurled

snake-like between
my parted lips

I am the not-remembering, a cracked glass sitting bereft on a shelf, having mastered the art of a smile so well no one can tell I can't tell who they are. ask me again if I remember and I can give another lie like a slice of lime, to cover the taste and pretend it's a feature. I'm a feature, a broken pen that only records some times, ink bruising the side of your hand. don't be angry; a glass is only a glass and cannot help its shatter. put me on a shelf and forget. that's what I'll do anyway. we could match. play twinsies. forget that forgetting is the ugly that stains you when a police officer asked you to ID the creep who broke into the mailbox and you say you can't. forget the betrayal in someone's eye when you forget their name again. forget the way a book ends. forget the worst things that happened—and the best.

the blue cup, whorling oil slick tan,
looking up from its shatter,
hears whisper   *shit*   understands.
so beautiful at shop this noon and now
in pieces, one lodging in foot, the closest it is to
becoming owner. it would bloodstream slip
into heart, brain, liver, to be close—
tweezers end dreams, even dreams of blue cup
fearing the night, not an hour owned
with perrier effervescence ticking
seconds away. not an hour
from lips sucking, hand grasping
entwining, caressing, dropping.
handled broom whispers final rites
across tiles. tool in owner's
fatal grasp ticks slivers softly into pan.
no drop of wine imbibed, no sugars
or stimulants served, cup bears
indignity in blue, staring as its
pricetag adheres to brown grout.

I wish I could be the person who calls CPS while everyone else sits on hands and laments, *Oh something is definitely wrong.* I would look you in the eyes even though you won't look into mine because that still makes you feel like someone will see too much of you or you will see too much of them. I would not touch you because I know you don't like to be touched, but I would say, *If you want a hug just let me know.* I would read your poetry and ignore your sister when she shoves drawings on top of the pages, and I would tell you that you will write truly great things one day, even if I know we never become the Next Greatest American Poet. I would comb your hair gently and ask what you'd like to do with it, and when you say you want to wear it short I would pull out scissors and give you the pixie cut mother never wanted us to have—I would make sure you don't wait another thirty years to feel that free. I would tell you that romance is overrated and that no one should ever touch you in a way you don't like, and when you started to tear up, I would open my arms and ask you to tell me what happened. I would listen and take you far, far away to a place where you would be loved and protected, where we could build the family we always should have had, and I would never let them lay a hand on you again.

you said I was two and I
                blank, grasp at the threads of
                        reality, learn anew what makes
                a person, what memories
build into. on your brown sofa I
                remember another couch
                        my therapist, *it's not*
                a full flashback and you
don't know when, it
                might not even be real
                        bed trembling, tonight
                my hands feel like not-my-hands
my skin needle-pricked
                and sweat-sensitive
                        you said you were so sorry
                for never telling anyone
while I try not to react, not to
                race my vomit to the toilet
                        not to tear-stream my terror
                tomorrow I will blank during
the drive, forget where I am
                rely on voice navigation
                        remember the times before
                GPS when I had to ask
gas station attendants
                what city I'm in, remember fear
                        of open highways and running
                out of gas, remember quaking
when the attendant is a man
                and I've never seen
                        this place before, remember the
                cold on a lonely 6 AM street
where a man followed me,

remember the click of his
heels on cold concrete. I swallow
swallow swallow, try to make
conversation, cling to strands of
thought as they slide past
I blank, I will have to ask
the girls what they just said
I pull out my phone, call
no one. and now I can
never be angry, can never
demand answers from
the military gravesite
you robbed me
of my chance for fury
for spitting fire, for sobbing
for feeling you feel my
pain. you said I was two
and I look into your eyes
feel myself disconnect, feel
the alien sensation, the skin
not my skin, in the throat
an unfamiliar calm
and I hear my voice say
it's okay.

Something unfolds
the splintered
branch its numerous self

petals violently
under the torrent
abundant pale

flesh breaks
into bronchioles
sucking the atmosphere

I lie awake trying
to remember the post
humous dreams of

where I left you

fish can become depressed, they say, the goldfish's
famous ten-second memory a hoax.

the pull between fish fantasy and fish reality blurs me,
unfurls the misunderstanding. I fish through memory,
count the angles of sadness on my fingers and toes
and rib bones and the ribbons I tie on each to remind.

because memory thinks it is funny, sending me for
the toilet paper I only remember ten seconds after
parking my grocery-laden car at home. is depression

the days huddled in one corner of a tank under covers
pretending this is life from now on. is it knowing
pain is what I get because it's what I deserve even when
I know it isn't, knowing how to hone an edge out of anything,
how to measure the stripes on my arm by the weather.
or maybe depression is spending ten hours playing a game
on my phone before deleting it.

how do they measure fish for hours of facebook lurking,
how do they measure the times fish check to see if anyone liked their post?
how many times did my goldfish write a letter he never intended to deliver?

once, I wrote an angry email and did not send it.
has my fish ever written an angry email and sent it accidentally?
on purpose? does he lie on an outstretched leaf, recalculating the events of
    the day?

the dosing for goldfish antidepressants must be done carefully,
homeopathically, diluted to the point of nontoxicity.
maybe I will swallow his dose, declare myself cured, write a book
about my ordeal, thank the scientists for their tireless effort
and the brave fish who paved the way.

There is gut-gnawing in lost time, the unconscious
posts to Twitter, logging on to FAFSA
only to discover financials I don't remember
entering, the journal I picked up—supposing it
empty—to find months of writing.
How many times did
my ex pull my hair, how often did
he kick me, did he push me to the
ground, body-slam me into a wall,
bruise my wrist? My teeth

have already lost their grounding.
Broken. I feel time pass retrospectively.
I check three clocks for lies—

a theater   the screen a black   and white movie
    a sigh   from the back rows   people
in the seats   lines of a poem   —   a staccato   of bodies
    a girl beside her sister   spits a hurricane   into the rows
pulls the seats   from their hardware   in the whirlwind   a house
    in the house   a father who   slinks outside
the bedroom door   outside the window   Dorothy's witch   watches sheets
    rise over   the bedframe   a road burns under

the broken home   a road of charcoal   bricks   the skeletal bracken
    a scarecrow   a tin man   a coward
are the girl's   father   they race her   to the emerald city
    the walls speak   softly   where her mother
projects   from her curtain   —   boom the voice

A sand crab crawls from the lapels of my grandfather's double-breasted suit, across prayerful hands, to the elbow and over silk lining his casket, from the edge, leaping onto seafoam carpet, another, then another, a wave of crustaceans, crawling over the lectern, over the feet of the priest, into barrels of rifles ready for the 21-gun salute, a crab crawls into my throat, I choke on the sea, my words eaten one by one, the little crab growing, it clambers into my lung, tiny stick feet poking and burning like liquid in my chest, my airways full of the sea, I cough and nothing comes up the way he coughed in the ER, the way he coughed while his lungs filled, the way he coughed when he told me the final secret, his loved ones crowd me, spit home remedies my way, ask me if I have forgiven my father yet, if I know how ill anger will make me as I try to swallow, try to cough, the ocean filling my thorax, grandfather told me he knew about the abuse when I was two, told me he was so sorry, he wished he had done something, said something, my heart pierced by an urchin's spiny body, leaking sea water, I pull myself through the crowd, a swimmer against rip tides, the crabs clawing my calves, my lungs burning I gasp for air, I make my way to my mother, my mother who sees my struggle, and—as always— she turns away.

the fallen tree branch—a sign from God
to sell your home
as bark tore moth wings from your arm.
did your body already know
the tearing within? the sick cells
replicating, replacing, fireflies
sparking alveoli, wild
lights at the edge of vision
and even when your vision failed the left eye,
you insisted on driving yourself,
drowning already, pneumatic
under the emergency room's crimson glare.
did your body feel a loop drawn tight
like a lasso around a fly's head?

I am not there to feel the chlorine in his lungs,
the tang of morphine in his gluteus
I imagine my grandfather's
cells bursting with chemo. I pray
without knowing what, liturgy seared onto
my lip. I burn pancakes again,
again I reach blindly for water, again
glass shards on the tile as I watch a dog piss
outside my window and wonder
at the yellow-painted crocuses
on the corner, burning in the ammonia.
I want to burn it all.

because the phone call came in just before noon,
and you wanted no measures to prolong your pain,
and I cried on a shoulder instead of rushing out the door,
and your son called and tried to dissuade me,
and there was unseasonable rain and traffic,
and I had to stop for gas halfway,
and I took the wrong offramp to avoid an accident,
and I had to make a U-turn to reach the after-hours entrance.

because they thought all the family had already left,
     the body was being wheeled to the morgue,
     the nurses, their voices,
     they forgot to pull the blanket to your throat,
     they forgot to uncurl your hands,
            unclench your jaw,
            lower your left eyelid,
            clean the spittle from your stubble.
     how cold the skin, how hard every line carved
     by the nasal cannula and its rubber tubing.

the rain was pouring, unseasonable, calling
to toadspawn asleep under cracked dirt
when the phone call came in before noon
under the rainfall spigot-open to full

spigot broken and emptying
over the dried mudswamp, they found you
unresponsive just before noon, the toadspawn
spontaneously generating their tails for a half hour

under the pour of the spigot, under
the drenched windshield, rainfall
laden with cracking and caked dirt splash-mixing
on the highway, the toadspawn
their tails, their waterlogged protolegs, mixed
into the mud under accident tires on the highway

the rainwater spigot-flowing over the windshield
the tadpoles breathing waterlogged mud under
the screeching tires, my car mud mixing
unresponsive toadspawn into gravel

under the spigot, the open emptying, the broken
emptying when the accident screech-wheel over
the mudswamp where tires ground tadpoles
their guts into mudthings

the spigotflow, pooled around swimming
toadspawn breathing mud and gravel, breathing in
the pour, breathing out the swimming

tadpoles breathing in their guts
the spigot open, I was open
under the spigot funnel and
the swimming toadspawn mud

and I was left open to full.

DEATH IS AN ACT OF CLEAVING

your gapped   lips   inhuman
without their teeth   like
a bird   humming in a bath   of dying
light, its beak   needles my   finger asleep
the hospital sign   its glow   a history
in relief   and the bird answers my call
plucks its down   nests with   longing
its honey-   guided tongue   caresses while
the not-you   waits   breathless
the not-you   its fingers   curled
the not-you   its mouth   a maw
a lump rises   and the bird asks   *can I*

time balances   on tiptoes   suspended
above Tucson   loss and
losing   red paint   chipping the edges

can I   the bird asks   and what
can I   answer

make me a vessel
I fill
with the dew

wash me in
a song of
stripped blades

of grass I will
myself to the earth
breathe green

waters float
my barren
breast I call

for the river
to tide
across my throat

reach my shores
I find no comfort
on the banks

of another
river drink deep
the blue heron

of the grass
blade lullaby
me to sleep

among reeds
bruised and
unbroken streams

the southward
song breaks into
clouds of dew

Rest on rocks naked
beside a dried-out Rio Grande.
I snake, I water-starve
I cacti-skin green and
hard. Hardy plants, dew
flowering through drought.
Monsoon winds cloud the sky
as I bake bone-dry and
aching. How I long for
the empty shells, their
infant feathers.
Once, I was pocked over
in clover, grew green
weeds and dandelion stems
and birds laid their eggs in a nest
of my hair.

i. waves

the waves
topple my bare
breasted stroke
falling into the blue

ii. creatures

octopus tendrils
leaving kiss marks
for someone to find
and question

puffer fish
beaking open
food, opening
skin, suckling
on blood borne
sustenance

iii. near death

chlorine
in waves, the ladder
cold and unattainable
my fingers
turning blue
like the plankton
phosphorescing in
tides, glowing
under moonlight

iv. mother ocean

the ocean laps
my released
breath
mother's face
drips into an expanse
of darkness
on that summer when
I breathed the blue
foam languishing
among seaweeds

v. lines in the sandy shore

little crabs
investigate the air
with bubbles, they crawl
along my
fingers when I reach
for the salt and wind,

I reach again for
the mother who birthed
the octopus, the secrets
that summer

she pulls off her eyelashes
first, sees how
to sew them doll-sensitive

and dark. she learns to
line the irises
in iridescents and the rest

is easy—the skin from
her thighs
a hearty blanket of wool

the heart and its muscles
standing on end
against her framework

wisps of flax dyed black
sewn with delicate
backstitch to the silk of

her crown. she holds
her breath
the last thread dangling

from her
unfinished pink lips

They meant no harm.

Is it intentions that matter now?

I am filleted   laid   bone-bare
and naked   on a block of wood
and here   an axe
slices   the clouds   from their perch
did I not   swim through
the canals and   craters   find
meaning in   upstream jaunts
swallow the green waters
inhale their   succulence   don't
pull my fins   from the roots
I am   here   to serve and be
served   on a platter   squeeze
lemon into the slit   in my side
rub salt into   my flesh I am
full of the rivers I will never
see again

I lost my ability
to fly. I twist
my folded body
into one position
too long, wake with

a crease along
my spine, the plain side
turned inward.

I grasp my ends, pull
myself into existence.

I can't remember like grandmother's
soap operas haunting the night
and in the morning a silhouette
on a pillow tidbits of paper
scrawls incoherent memory
I struggle for a word on the very tip
willing to plunge head-first and fast
places with no names attached
or into the arms of strangers
how deeply the writing is locked behind
a glass door on a shelf
I read a book in my own hand

APPENDIX

POEMS THAT PREVIOUSLY APPEARED IN OTHER PUBLICATIONS

PACIFIC REVIEW:"Things I Learned from my Mother"

[ISACOUSTIC]: "A Longing For" and "you heard his voice in"

[ISACOUSTIC]:"For Love" (now "Ars Poetica")

RIGGWELTER:"Mother Musing Over Her Daughter's Doll"

TYPEHOUSE:"Climate Change"

EUNOIA REVIEW:"Visiting Grandfather on my Way to New Mexico,"
"Into the Blue," "Cupboards," "Mother Musing Over Her Daughter's
Doll," and "Mother Musing Over the Daughter's Doll"

DARK ONUS LIT:"Nothing Green Grows in the Desert," "do not tell
me we are," and "Swan Song"

THE JOURNAL OF RADICAL WONDER: "Nothing green grows
in the desert," "15 minutes late," "A Lament from Ghosts," "the
subtle longing," "Desert Mythology," "Ars Poetica," "Sisterhood,"
"Bathtime," "The Owl," and "Semi-Precious"

NOTES ON VARIOUS POEMS IN THIS MANUSCRIPT

page 14 "First We Make the Beast Beautiful" is the title of a
2018 New York Times Bestselling Book by Sarah Wilson about living
with anxiety

page 20 This quote by Kyle Hill is from his June 25, 2013
Scientific American article titled, "The Fungus that Reduced
Humanity to The Last of Us"

page 21 In "Desert Mythology," the line "Inside, one bowl
fills another" borrows wording and cadence from Connie Voisine's
poem, "This World and That One"

page 28 This epigraph reflects an August 9, 2018 Washington
Post article by Emily Wax-Thibodeaux titled, "This place 'is going to
burn,' says text allegedly sent by man arrested in California's Holy
Fire"

page 30 This epigraph and text within this poem
    reflect quotes by firefighting representatives regarding
    the Holy Fire, used in the above-referenced August 9,
    2018 Washington Post article

page 32 This catalog of photographs reflects the
    images paired with the above-referenced August 9,
    2018 Washington Post article

page 40 This poem obliquely references an
    October 16, 2017 New York Times article by Heather
    Murphy titled, "Fish Depression Is Not A Joke," which
    recounts how Dr. Julian Pittman and other researchers
    test the efficacy of antidepressant medication on fish

page 49 "Swan Song" is an elegy heavily inspired
    by Chad Sweeney's Little Million Doors, which itself
    is an elegy to his father

ABOUT THE AUTHOR

Tiffany Elliott is an asexual, neuroatypical, and disabled woman and mental health professional who received her MFA from New Mexico State University. Her debut collection, *Bones Awaiting the Blaze*, was awarded the 2022 Hillary Gravendyk Prize, and her work has appeared in *Typehouse, Spectrum*, and other journals. Her works explore the mythologies we experience, those we create for ourselves, issues of abuse and trauma, and how people can remake themselves.

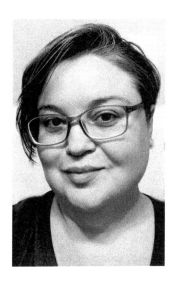

ABOUT INLANDIA INSTITUTE

Inlandia Institute is a regional non-profit and literary center. We seek to bring focus to the richness of the literary enterprise that has existed in this region for ages. The mission of the Inlandia Institute is to recognize, support, and expand literary activity in all of its forms in Inland Southern California by publishing books and sponsoring programs that deepen people's awareness, understanding, and appreciation of this unique, complex and creatively vibrant region.

The Institute publishes books, presents free public literary and cultural programming, provides in-school and after school enrichment programs for children and youth, holds free creative writing workshops for teens and adults, and boot camp intensives. In addition, every two years, the Inlandia Institute appoints a distinguished jury panel from outside of the region to name an Inlandia Literary Laureate who serves as an ambassador for the Inlandia Institute, promoting literature, creative literacy, and community. Laureates to date include Susan Straight (2010-2012), Gayle Brandeis (2012-2014), Juan Delgado (2014-2016), Nikia Chaney (2016-2018), and Rachelle Cruz (2018-2020).

To learn more about the Inlandia Institute, please visit our website at www.InlandiaInstitute.org.

ABOUT THE HILLARY GRAVENDYK PRIZE

The Hillary Gravendyk Prize is an open poetry book competition published by Inlandia Institute for all writers regardless of the number of previously published poetry collections.

HILLARY GRAVENDYK (1979-2014) was a beloved poet living and teaching in Southern California's "Inland Empire" region. She wrote the acclaimed poetry book, *HARM* from Omnidawn Publishing (2012) and the posthumoussly published *The Soluble Hour* (Omnidawn, 2017) and *Unlikely Conditions* (1913 Press, 2017, with Cynthia Arrieu-King) as well as the poetry chapbook *The Naturalist* (Anchiote Press, 2008). A native of Washington State, she was an admired Assistant Professor of English at Pomona College in Claremont, CA. Her poetry has appeared widely in journals such as *American Letters & Commentary*, *The Bellingham Review*, *The Colorado Review*, *The Eleventh Muse*, *Fourteen Hills*, *MARY*, *1913: A Journal of Forms*, *Octopus Magazine*, *Tarpaulin Sky and Sugar House Review*. She was awarded a 2015 Pushcart Prize for her poem "Your Ghost," which appeared in the Pushcart Prize Anthology. She leaves behind many devoted colleagues, friends, family and beautiful poems. Hillary Gravendyk passed away on May 10, 2014 after a long illness. This contest has been established in her memory.

OTHER HILLARY GRAVENDYK PRIZE BOOKS

the artemisia by William S. Barnes
Winner of the 2022 National Hillary Gravendyk Prize

How To Know You're Dreaming When You're Dreaming, Lesson One
    by Angelica Maria Barraza Tran
Winner of the 2021 National Hillary Gravendyk Prize

Our Lady of Perpetual Desert by Alexandra Martinez
Winner of the 2021 Regional Hillary Gravendyk Prize

among the enemies by Michael Samra
Winner of the 2020 Regional Hillary Gravendyk Prize

This Side of the Fire by Jonathan Maule
Winner of the 2020 Regional Hillary Gravendyk Prize

The Silk the Moths Ignore by Bronwen Tate
Winner of the 2019 National Hillary Gravendyk Prize

Remyth: A Postmodern Ritual by Adam D. Martinez
Winner of the 2019 Regional Hillary Gravendyk Prize

Former Possessions of the Spanish Empire by Michelle Peñaloza
Winner of the 2018 National Hillary Gravendyk Prize

All the Emergency-Type Structures by Elizabeth Cantwell
Winner of the 2018 Regional Hillary Gravendyk Prize

Our Bruises Kept Singing Purple by Malcolm Friend
Winner of the 2017 National Hillary Gravendyk Prize

Traces of a Fifth Column by Marco Maisto
Winner of the 2016 National Hillary Gravendyk Prize

God's Will for Monsters by Rachelle Cruz
Winner of the 2016 Regional Hillary Gravendyk Prize
Winner of a 2018 American Book Award

Map of an Onion by Kenji C. Liu
Winner of the 2015 National Hillary Gravendyk Prize

All Things Lose Thousands of Times by Angela Peñaredondo
Winner of the 2015 Regional Hillary Gravendyk Prize

Printed in the USA
CPSIA information can be obtained
at www.ICGtesting.com
LVHW021332270424
778630LV00011BA/524